ACID REFLUX DIET COOKBOOK

Tasty Acid Reflux Recipes to Prevent Heartburn Problems

(Curing Your Indigestion by Taking Diets Free of Gluten and Acidic Composition)

Kristine Aleman

Published by Alex Howard

© **Kristine Aleman**

All Rights Reserved

Acid Reflux Diet Cookbook: Tasty Acid Reflux Recipes to Prevent Heartburn Problems (Curing Your Indigestion by Taking Diets Free of Gluten and Acidic Composition)

ISBN 978-1-77485-005-3

Legal & Disclaimer

The information contained in this book is not designed to replace or take the place of any form of medicine or professional medical advice. The information in this book has been provided for educational and entertainment purposes only.

Table of contents

Part 1

1

Introduction

Acid reflux is an increasingly common condition today as our lifestyles and eating habits have deteriorated. In the United States, over 60 million people experience acid reflux at least once a month and about 15 million Americans experience heartburn on a daily basis. This is based on a report issued by the American College of Gastroenterology.

Westerners are more likely to have heartburn compared to their Asian counterparts. Approximately one in five Americans who have acid reflux and one in six Americans have the risk factors to develop it.

Acid reflux is often referred to in simpler terms as heartburn because of the pain felt around and below the chest, which is often mistaken as a symptom of heart disease. It happens when the acid from the stomach goes back to the esophagus as there is a blockage or abnormality in the gastroesophageal sphincter.

This medical condition is one of the most popular searches on the Internet, as most people are not aware of its causes and the possible complications such as cancer of the throat and esophagus. The causes of acid reflux may differ from one person to another. It is advisable that sufferers see a doctor to receive a proper diagnosis and treatment plan, rather than administering self-medication such as pain killers or antacids on their own as they may have side-effects later on.

This book contains proven steps and strategies on how to prevent and treat acid reflux and gastroesophageal reflux disease (GERD) by learning the different diet strategies, home remedies, foods to eat and to avoid, and advice on post acid reflux gastrointestinal health.

Also discussed in this book are alternative therapies and traditional therapies. You will learn the basics, causes, symptoms, diagnosing, lifestyle changes, and treatment options for this medical condition to enable you to manage it and prevent its discomfort and complications.

Thanks again for downloading my book, I hope you enjoy it!

Chapter 1: Understanding Acid Reflux

Acid reflux is a medical condition that is associated with flowing up of the stomach acid, which is mostly composed of hydrochloric acid, into the food pipe or esophagus. In some people the acid reflux comes in between burping, which can be embarrassing especially when eating in public.

The hydrochloric acid aids in the proper food digestion and acts as protector from bacteria. Our stomach is a complex organ that is composed of various parts. Its lining is designed to produce the acid that protects the digestive tract system against wear and tear, particularly from ulcers when there is not enough food to digest as well as combatting H. pylori infection.

What Is H. pylori?

Helicobacter pylorus is a bacterium that may invade the body and dwell in the digestive tract. Their presence is not easily felt as they slowly harm the gastrointestinal tract by causing sores or ulcer. Some infection caused by H. pylori may cause ulcers, bleeding and cancer and some may cause other symptoms. There are medications available to kill the bacteria and cure the ulcer. The bacteria come from poor sanitation and contaminated water.

Facts about Acid Reflux:

There are many things that every person should know about acid reflux that most people are unaware of. Here are the facts:

1. It has many names such as GERD or gastroesophageal reflux disease and heartburn. It is also called as acid indigestion or pyrosis.
2. The condition will be called GERD when the symptoms of acid reflux happen more than twice per week.
3. It is a common ailment among Westerners, particularly Americans.
4. The esophagus is protected by gastroesophageal sphincter, which is composed of muscle, from possible harm brought about by the stomach contents. The muscle acts as a gate valve by blocking the stomach entrance.
5. Heartburn happens when there is an abnormal activity in the gastroesophageal sphincter, where the acid from the stomach flows up into the esophagus or food pipe.
6. It is commonly felt after eating and accompanied with burning pain around or below the chest area.
7. Smoking and obesity can trigger acid reflux.
8. It is treatable with over-the-counter medications and alternative medicine.
9. GERD can lead to complications and the most feared is cancer.
10. Heartburn has nothing to do with the heart, although the pain is below or around the chest area.

11. A sour or bitter taste in the throat and mouth can be felt for a few minutes to hours.
12. Spitting more often by chewing a gum helps a lot to swallow more acid and push the acid back to the stomach.
13. Sleeping with pillows on top of another can relieve you of heartburn.
14. Wearing tight jeans and sleeping after eating can trigger heartburn.
15. It usually occurs after eating, sleeping after eating and physical activity after eating.

Prevalence of Acid Reflux:

Based on the report made by the American College of Gastroenterology, acid reflux is one of the most common illnesses in the United States. Sixty million Americans can experience heartburn once in a month.

Fifteen million Americans have symptoms of acid reflux almost every day. To sum up, about 20 to 30% of the populations in Western countries are suffering from this condition.

About one in five Americans are prone to have heartburn and one in 6 Americans have high risks of acid reflux, or 40 % of the adult population. Its prevalence has increased about 50% from ten years ago in the Norwegian population based on a report issued by the medical journal "Gut" in the last quarter of 2011.

Causes of Acid Reflux:

Acid reflux may occur once in a blue moon to some people and others experience it frequently. The discomfort is usually accompanied with pain right below the breastbone area, which may cause you to panic. It can happen to anyone, regardless of age, but more common among Caucasians, for reasons remain unknown.

It can be caused by:

1. Lifestyle factors such as obesity and smoking.
2. Hiatal hernia-This is an abnormality in the human anatomy where the chest cavity is pushed by the upper section of the stomach through the entrance of the diaphragm or hiatus. When there is a hiatal hernia, the sufferer will experience frequent acid reflux because of the bulges in the stomach that is going in the direction of the chest cavity.
3. Pregnancy-In some cases, the acid my flow back to the esophagus as the baby bump is getting bigger.
4. Physical inactivity
5. High sodium intake
6. Low intake of dietary fiber-Fiber can neutralize the acid in the stomach and it aids in proper digestion of food.
7. Taking medications to treat existing ailments such as antidepressant drugs, sedatives, antihistamines, ibuprofen, and calcium-channel blockers.

8. Drinking alcohol, carbonated and caffeinated beverages.
9. Eating close to bedtime or eating a heavy meal before bedtime
10. Lying down and bending over after a meal.
11. Eating foods that can trigger heartburn.
12. Wearing tight clothes, belts and pants.

Symptoms of Acid Reflux:

- You will taste something bitter and sour in the throat and mouth after a meal, lying down or stooping.
- Stomach bloating
- Frequent burping
- In rare cases, bloody vomit or black stools
- Hiccups
- Nausea
- Food stuck in the throat called dysphagia
- Wheezing
- Dry cough
- Hoarseness of voice
- Persistent sore throat
- Discomfort and burning pain right below the breastbone area and sometimes reaches the throat area.

Who are at risk of acid reflux?

Acid reflux may occur at any age. Children can have it at a younger age and some may experience heartburn as they grow older. You are at risk if you have any of the following:

- If you are obese
- If you are pregnant
- If you love to wear tight-fitting clothes, pants and belts
- If you have hiatal hernia
- If you are a passive or active smoker
- If you have sedentary life
- If you have low fiber diet
- If you love spicy and irritating foods
- If you eat close to bedtime
- If you are fond of salty foods

Complications of acid reflux:

Acid reflux can lead to complications if it is uncontrolled and left untreated. Both esophagitis and Barrett's esophagus may lead to cancer in some patients. This is based on a 1999 study that was reported in the New England Journal of Medicine.

The study disclosed the connection between cancer and acid reflux. Patients are therefore advised to seek medical advice if their condition persists even after taking medications and applying home remedies.

In recent studies by the American Association for Cancer Research in 2013, it reported that there is a big possibility that untreated acid reflux may lead to cancers of the throat and the vocal cord. The same study said that antacids can help a lot in controlling acidity in the stomach.

When the symptoms of acid reflux persist within a week it will develop into GERD or gastroesophageal reflux disease resulting in more serious medical problems such as:

1. Barrett's esophagus-This is a serious illness that is caused by chronic GERD. It can also occur in people who do not have GERD, but generally it can be a risk factor for Barrett's esophagus. Acid reflux can be the cause of Barrett's esophagus if it happens many times that lead to abnormalities in the cells that are found in the esophageal lining. The damaged cell will then be replaced with an unusual type of cells in the esophagus putting the patient at risk of cancer. In some cases, not all people with Barrett's esophagus will lead to cancer.

2. Esophagitis- This condition is accompanied with irritation and pain in the esophagus due to backwash of the stomach acid. This is the result of pressure in the esophageal lining when the acid keeps on going back to the esophagus causing ulceration, scarring and bleeding. People who have esophagitis are at risk of getting cancer.

3. Esophageal bleeding-There are many causes of esophageal bleeding, among them is liver scarring. Chronic liver disease may result in bleeding that overflows to the esophageal lining, causing esophageal varices or enlargement of the veins. Aside from liver disease, stomach varices due to duodenal scarring and stomach acidity may also result to bleeding that needs prompt medical attention.

4. Ulcers-Acid reflux may develop into a painful sore in the gastrointestinal and esophageal linings. It happens when the lining becomes eroded because of constant pressure by the acid. Untreated stomach ulcers may become malignant. If you are having abdominal pain that do not stop, seek medical attention as soon as possible.

5. Esophageal cancer-When acid reflux become frequent it will develop into a GERD causing irritation and bleeding in the esophagus as the stomach acid keeps on flowing back. Cancer growth starts from the cells in the esophageal lining.

6. Strictures-They are injuries caused by acid reflux because of the pressure of constant flowing of acid into the esophagus. The acid will result to inflammation and scarring in the esophagus. Sufferers may have a hard time swallowing their food as they can feel the irritation when the food is stuck while traveling to the esophagus.

This chapter has been dedicated to the basics of acid reflux, causes and symptoms, to inform readers that this medical condition should be treated to avoid complications. In succeeding chapters, you will learn the different tests and exams to diagnose acid reflux, homeopathy, alternative medicine, surgical options, and postoperative care after surgery and dietary plan. Each chapter will give you full details about the different approaches, strategies and advices on how to deal with acid reflux and to prevent its complications to your body as well as food recommendations to have a regular bowel movements.

Chapter 2: Diagnosing Acid Reflux

Acid reflux is not a serious illness if it only happens once in a month as most individuals may experience it at some points of their lives. It may happen if they go to bed immediately after they eat dinner or stoop down.

When the symptoms of acid reflux happen more than two times per week, it becomes a GERD or gastroesophageal reflux disease that could lead to complications, even if all treatments have been applied.

Physical examination is needed this time if there is no lasting relief, even if you have employed lifestyle changes and home remedies. The doctor will order several tests to diagnose the real causes of acid reflux and check if there are underlying causes of the discomfort.

Types of Tests for Acid Reflux:

1. Monitoring of pH-This is performed by the doctor to check the acidity of the esophagus by inserting a device to the patient's esophagus and allow it to stay for one to two days. This is to determine the pH level of the gut flora in the digestive tract.
2. Endoscopy-The doctor will look inside the patient's esophagus and gastrointestinal tract with the use of

an endoscope. The patient has to empty the bowel and refrain from taking solids several hours before performing the endoscopy. The doctor or surgeon will sedate the patient using a general anesthesia to avoid discomfort.

3. Barium swallow-Before performing this test, the doctor will let the patient swallow barium sulfate solution to have a vivid X-ray examination of the upper gastrointestinal tract. This is to check if the patient has narrow esophagus or have stomach problems. The barium sulfate is mixed with water and once ingested by the patient; it coats the intestinal walls and lining of the stomach to have a clearer picture of what is happening inside.

4. Biopsy-This is to check the tissue samples taken from the gastrointestinal tract and esophagus while performing an endoscopy. The doctor will check the specimen using a microscope to see for possible anatomical abnormalities and infection inside the body.

5. Esophageal manometry-This test is used to measure the muscle coordination and the strength of the esophagus when the patient is swallowing food. A tube is inserted into the nose that will pass the throat, and then to the esophagus and lastly into the stomach. Manometry is performed to patients who have symptoms of acid reflux or heartburn by observing the peristalsis of the esophagus.

Peristalsis is the movement of the muscles in the esophagus, particularly the esophageal sphincter, which is a muscular valve that opens when the food passes and closes to discourage the food and the stomach acid from moving out of the stomach and then going up to the esophagus. Pregnant women and individuals with lung, heart and other chronic ailments should tell their doctor prior to the esophageal manometry.

6. Esophageal impedance-pH monitoring-This outpatient test is performed to measure the non-acid reflux and acidity of the stomach contents by placing the sensors in the esophagus. The patient wears a data recorder by which the symptomatic episodes are recorded for analysis and find out if it is related to the reflux episodes. This test is usually performed within 24 hours. The patient is advised to empty the bowel and avoid eating or drinking four hours prior to the test.

When to seek medical help?

Sufferers of GERD, heartburn or acid reflux should seek professional help if the medications and home remedies are ineffective. It signals that a specialist in gastroenterology should check your medical condition to have the right treatment administered and prevent complications.

It is time to seek medical help if you have any of the following:

- If you have chest pain.
- If it is accompanied by shortness of breath.
- Pain that reaches the arm and jaw.
- If the bleeding and pain persist.
- If your voice is hoarse.
- If you have difficulty in swallowing your food.
- If the symptoms of heartburn is more than twice in a week.
- If the medications and prevention techniques are ineffective.
- If you lost your voice.

Preparing for an appointment:

Acid reflux is not dangerous initially, but when it develops into a gastroesophageal reflux disease, complications may arise. When the symptoms continue after taking antacids and proton-pump inhibitors (PPIs), you have to seek professional help. Be prepared to answer and ask questions to your doctor. Use the FAQs below as reference when consulting your doctor.

Here are frequently asked questions by patients:

1. What are the possible causes of acid reflux?
2. Are there other ailments that have caused my condition?

3. What are the tests needed to diagnose my condition?

4. Which test is best for my age and my existing health condition?

5. What medications should I take?

6. Are these medications safe for my health?

7. What are the complications if I will not take oral medications?

8. What are the side-effects of taking anti-reflux medications?

9. What is the right treatment other than taking medications?

10. Is surgery suitable for my age?

11. What causes relapse or recurrence of GERD after a surgery?

12. I am pregnant, what treatment is best for my condition?

13. How much is the cost of surgery?

14. What is the best diet for me?

FAQ from a health professional:

- How many times the symptoms occur in a week?
- Is it accompanied with bleeding and burning pain?
- Do you smoke?
- Do you eat a high fiber diet?
- Are your meals spicy and fatty?
- Do you have chest pain?
- Does the pain reach the arm, jaw and shoulders?

- Do you lie down or exercise after eating?
- Do you have difficulty swallowing your food?
- What medications are you taking?

Health professionals to look for:

- Gastroenterologist
- Internist
- Family medicine doctor
- Surgeon
- Nurse
- Nurse assistant
- Pharmacist

The muscles found in the lower part of the esophageal sphincter normally opens to allow the food to pass from the throat down to the stomach and automatically close to discourage the stomach acids from slipping into the esophagus. When the function of the esophageal sphincter becomes abnormal because of underlying issues, the acid from the stomach will slide up into the esophageal lining and the throat, which release a sour and bitter tasting fluid.

In some people, the acids are so prevalent that they are hardly able to breathe for a few seconds. The pain can be felt in the lower part of the chest area and this is where heartburn takes place. It should be noted that not all cases of acid reflux can lead to heartburn or if there is heartburn that is accompanied with shortness of breath and chest pain, it may signal another disease that should not be overlooked by the sufferer.

Chapter 3: Prevention & Treatment For Acid Reflux

There are many ways to prevent acid reflux and gastroesophageal reflux disease that sufferers can employ. Lifestyle factors can contribute to the progression of acid reflux to become a full blown gastroesophageal reflux disease (GERD) that will ultimately lead to complications and even cancer. Prevention is very important to avoid this condition; among them is a lifestyle change. Obesity and smoking are said to be the primary causes of acid reflux and need to be countered at its onset.

Tips on preventing acid reflux:

- Try to lose weight by controlling your diet and proper exercise.
- Stop smoking.
- Increase your intake of high fiber diet.
- Do not sleep right after taking your meals.
- Minimize eating salty, fatty and spicy foods.
- Keep a diary or journal to trace its causes.
- Avoid drinking alcohol, caffeinated and carbonated drinks.
- Eat small, frequent meals.
- Refrain from exercises that require you to sit up or bend after a meal.
- Add more pillows to elevate your head.
- Sleep in a chair when having a daytime nap.

- Avoid wearing tight jeans, belts and clothes.
- Refer to your doctor if you are taking other medications that might trigger the acid reflux symptoms.

Medications for Acid Reflux:

There are many medications that patients can take to relieve the symptoms of acid reflux and most of them do not need a doctor's prescription. These medications include proton pump inhibitors or PPIs and antacids to reduce stomach acidity, and ibuprofen to remove the burning pain caused by heartburn and GERD.

Proton-Pump Inhibitors and Acid Reflux:

Acid reflux is a treatable disease but may develop into a complicated illness, such as cancer. At the onset of this condition, the sufferer may choose to take proton-pump inhibitors or PPIs. PPI is a type of drugs that help reduce acid production in the stomach to prevent ulcers, hyperacidity, gastritis and acid reflux. PPIs block the enzymes in the intestinal wall where the acid is produced.

Acid is the main agent in developing ulceration and scarring in the gastrointestinal tract and esophagus. Long-term use of proton pump inhibitor medications should be stopped if the symptoms of acid reflux persist as it can cause organ damage, blocks the absorption of nutrients, infection risk and among others. The PPIs can be bought as over-the-counter medication and it has been commercially available for more than two decades now.

List of Proton-Pump Inhibitors (PPIs):

1. Protonix (pantoprazole)-It is prescribed as a treatment for esophagitis and Zollinger-Ellison syndrome and acid reflux because of its ability to reduce stomach acid. Patients with history of allergies in certain medications such as pantoprazole and benzimidazole, as well as illnesses such as liver disease, osteoporosis, osteopenia and low magnesium in the blood should ask their doctor for advice.
2. Aciphex (rabeprazole) –This oral medication is used to reduce stomach acidity that causes acid reflux and GERD. It is also used to heal duodenal and esophageal ulcers, Zollinger-Ellison syndrome, and H. pylori infections. It can be taken both on an empty or filled stomach.
3. Nexium (esomeprazole) -This PPI helps reduce the amount of stomach acid to treat gastroesophageal reflux disease or acid reflux, Zollinger-Ellison syndrome, erosive esophagitis and prevent bleeding in the esophagus. It can be taken orally or injected when the patient cannot take it by mouth.
4. Prevacid (lansoprazole)-It reduces the acid production in the stomach and treats erosive esophagitis and intestinal ulcers.

5. Dexilant (dexlansoprazole)-This oral medication is used to treat acid reflux, GERD and prevents esophageal ulcers and bleeding by reducing the amount of acid in the stomach. Consult a doctor if symptoms of GERD persist even after long-term use.
6. Egerid (immediate-release omeprazole with sodium bicarbonate)
7. Prilosec & Zegerid (omeprazole)-It is prescribed by a gastroenterologist to reduce the stomach acid, treat GERD and erosive esophagitis. For patients with gastric ulcer caused by H. pylori infection, can take omeprazole along with antibiotics.

Antacids and Gastric Reflux:

People who are prone to have dyspepsia, hyperacidity and acid reflux can also take antacids to neutralize stomach acid triggered by missed meals and drinking alcoholic beverages. They can buy antacids without a doctor's prescription as they are commercially available in chewable tablets, chewing gum, dissolving tablets, and liquid forms from pharmacies. They are taken to alleviate the pain and acidity by reacting with the contents of the stomach and not directly on the cells that produce acids in the duodenal lining.

Antacids are composed of various compounds that include magnesium hydrochloride, aluminum, sodium bicarbonate and calcium carbonate. Although antacids are generally safe to use for pregnant and lactating women, it is not recommended for children under 12 years old and for patients with kidney disease. Mild cases of acid reflux and GERD can be remedied with antacids, but taking it for more than two weeks is not advisable.

Types of Antacids:

- Calcium carbonate - They come with brand names Tums and Rolaids, which promotes absorption of calcium in the body.
- Aluminum hydroxide & magnesium carbonate - They come with a brand name Gaviscon, which is composed of alginic acid and foaming agent. The top of the stomach contents will be coated with the antacid to prevent the acid from direct contact with the esophagus. The alginate is derived from brown algae.
- Aluminum hydroxide & magnesium hydroxide - They come with brand names Maalox and Mylanta that have simethicone, which is responsible in breaking down the air inside the stomach. Flatulence and burping are reduced after taking this medication.

Other Medications and Acid Reflux:

There are certain medications to treat other ailments that can trigger the symptoms of acid reflux. Among them are pain killers, antidepressants, antibiotics, nitroglycerin, and drugs for the treatment of anxiety, hypertension and osteoporosis.

It is understood that if you have hypertension and psychosomatic illness, stopping their medication can make your existing condition worse. If you want to remove the discomfort of acid reflux, you have to inform your doctor about your other medications to avoid contraindications and side effects. You may still have to take all your medications on a certain schedule. Here are some facts on how to address this problem:

- Read the medical literature and check the instructions carefully.
- You should be aware that there are certain drugs that are to be taken before or after meals.
- Not following the instruction can only worsen your health condition.
- Do not take more than what your doctor recommends.
- Follow the schedule of all your medications and do not double dose for a missed schedule.
- Avoid self-medication to treat acid reflux, especially if you have another illness.
- Post your doctor's prescription and schedule of medications in a cork board.

Reminders when taking medications:

Note that antacids should not be taken in combination with proton pump inhibitors, or taken within one hour of each other as the antacid has the ability to slow down the function of PPIs. Although PPI is prescribed to block the acid in the stomach, over dosage may cause the stomach to produce less acid.

In his editorial, San Francisco Department of Public Health chief Mitchell Katz pointed out that PPIs does not at all guarantee to treat GERD, heartburn and acid reflux because their functions are only limited in the treatment of bleeding ulcers, Zollinger-Ellison syndrome, and severe case of acid reflux.

Katz added that the dependence of PPIs will decrease the body's natural ability to block the H. pylori bacteria because the stomach acid is depleted. Stomach acid serves as a blocking force against bacterial infection that may cause food poisoning. The PPIs can trigger bone loss, hip fracture and pulmonary infection.

Melatonin and Acid Reflux:

Melatonin is an indole that is said to cause sleep. Melatonin plays a major role in stimulating the activity of the lower esophageal sphincter so that stomach contents will not back up into the esophagus. This conclusion is based on animal studies as reported by the Life Extension Foundation.

Melatonin has been proven effective in healing sores and ulcers in the digestive tract. Its presence in the GI tract through the enterochromaffin cells can prevent and cure irritable bowel syndrome, stomach upset and dyspepsia. Taking melatonin along with natural food supplements are more effective compared to proton pump inhibitors, particularly omeprazole.

Chapter 4: Natural Remedies For Acid Reflux

Whatever it is, whether it is acid reflux or Gerd, this medical condition can cause discomfort to the sufferer. It happens when the acid from the stomach goes back to the throat or esophagus. When it occurs, a mixture of sour and bitter taste fluid seem to block the breast and throat areas. Sometimes it can make the sufferer panic when they are unable to inhale air because of the blockage.

Burping and expelling gas from the anus may seem to relieve the symptoms. There is no other remedy that the sufferer may think of at that time, except to take over-the-counter medications; the most common are antacids and painkillers. But what if the heartburn continues for a couple of days, then the condition may develop into GERD or gastroesophageal reflux disease. At that time is has to be referred to a specialist.

Prolonged use of antacids can have adverse effects on your health. Why not try using home remedies that are proven and tested to alleviate acid reflux, if not totally remove the symptoms. There are many products that are available in the market to relieve GERD, heartburn and acid reflux. If you scrutinize their contents, most of them are concoctions from the fruit, leaves, bark and roots of trees, shrubs and herbal plants.

Here is a rundown of some common home remedies:

1. Iberis amara-Candytuft is known for its medicinal properties to treat gout, rheumatism, asthma, bronchitis and to aid in food digestion. The seeds are more effective in reducing acidity in the stomach. It should be taken moderately to avoid diarrhea, nausea and giddiness.

2. Angelica radix-Aside from its culinary uses, angelica root is used for medicinal purposes; among them is reduction of gastric acid secretion in the stomach.

3. Silybum mariani fructus-Milk thistle extracts are known as liver tonics and they are used as a treatment for gallbladder disorder and reduction of acidity in the stomach.

4. Apple cider vinegar-Take one tablespoon of apple cider vinegar with a full glass of water to neutralize the stomach acidity.

5. Baking soda-Sodium bicarbonate is one of the main ingredients in drugs to treat stomach upset, hyperacidity and acid reflux. Take one half to one teaspoon with a glass of water to neutralize stomach acidity.

6. Aloe juice-Aloe vera has many uses in medicine such as relieving inflammation caused by burn and other bodily ailments, including acid reflux. To neutralize acidity, drink one half of aloe juice, one hour before meals for proper absorption.

7. Betaine-There are betaine supplements available in health food stores and pharmacies. Look for betaine

hydrochloric supplement and they come in capsule or liquid form. Betaine acts in proper food digestion and maintaining the gut flora of the stomach by killing the H. pylori bacteria.

8. Glutamine   This amino acid is effective in treating acid reflux or GERD by neutralizing the stomach acid and control the H. pylori infection. Glutamine is found in dairy products, fruits, vegetable and meat and in food supplements.

9. Folic acid or Vitamin B9-This nutrient is essential in the reduction of acid reflux with 40% efficacy. Food sources of folic acid are from legumes, beans, spinach, okra, asparagus and liver.

10. Ulmus rubra-The bark and leaves of slippery elm are used in concocting tea to soothe the gastrointestinal tract, mouth and throat. It helps alleviate acid reflux by neutralizing stomach acidity and bowel disorder. Pregnant women are discouraged from taking Ulmus rubra tea. Boil 2 tablespoons of pulverized slippery elm bark with 2 cups of water for about five minutes. Drink the tea three times a day.

11. Zingiber officinale-Ginger root is effective in blocking stomach acid and controlling H. pylori infection in the stomach. Ginger ale can soothe the stomach and throat and it is effective in removing gas pain, and prevents ulceration in the esophagus and intestine. Boil three slices of ginger root in two glasses of water for 10 minutes or until the mixture

becomes brownish. Drink the ginger ale as soon as you wake up or before meals.

12. Chamomile-It is used for treating depression, insomnia, and generalized anxiety disorder. Its anti-inflammatory properties are effective in treating hemorrhoids and gastrointestinal and esophageal inflammation. For effective use in treating acid reflux, drink a cup of chamomile tea before bedtime.

13. Vitamin D-High intake of vitamin D can increase the production of antimicrobial peptides that helps prevents inflammation and infection in the body, among them is your stomach and esophagus. There are Vitamin D supplements available in health food stores and you can get ample amount by having sun exposure early in the morning.

14. Astaxanthin-It is an antioxidant with a reddish pigmentation found in algae, shrimps, lobsters, crabs and trouts. It is proven to be effective in the treatment of brain disorders such as stroke, Alzheimer's disease, macular degeneration and Parkinson's disease. As an antioxidant, it has the ability to protect the cells in the body against damage and reduction of acidity in the stomach especially in combatting H. pylori infection. For effective use, take a dose of 40 milligrams of astaxanthin daily.

15. Licorice-This plant is used in the manufacturing of beauty and cosmetic products, tobacco and

beverages. It is also used in cooking and when it comes to medicine, it can prevent and cure acid reflux, colitis, gastritis, hyperacidity and stomach ulcers. Other ailments can be treated with licorice includes tuberculosis, lupus, liver diseases, osteoarthritis, malaria, chronic fatigue syndrome and food poisoning.

16. Caraway-This plant is used in enhancing food flavors and known for its medicinal properties. Women use its oil to have regular menstruation, removes dysmenorrhea and increase milk production after childbirth. Caraway is used in cooking as food enhancer. It is also used to relieve cough, constipation, stomach upset and acid reflux.

17. Lemon balm-The leaves of lemon balm are used to relieve pain caused by menstrual cramps, upset stomach, toothache, headache, flatulence, colic, vomiting and acid reflux. Drink a cup of lemon balm tea, if you are having symptoms of heartburn and GERD at least three times a day. Lemon balm has calming effects in the body, especially in patients suffering from anxiety, nervousness, depression, ADHD, and other mental disorders.

18. Orange peel-GERD sufferers can take orange peel extracts in capsule form sold at drug stores. For effective results, they should take it thrice a week or until the symptoms of reflux subside. If you have oranges at home, do not throw the peel, use it as a remedy for acid reflux.

19. Coconut-Fresh coconut water is known for its therapeutic properties as it can prevent kidney disease. Drink fresh coconut water early in the morning before breakfast or as often as you want to remove the symptoms of acid reflux or GERD. For a start, you drink about eight ounces of coconut water with three teaspoons of coconut oil and drink it slowly.

20. Almonds-They are not only great in making desserts, they are useful in the prevention and cure of acid reflux. Eat almonds daily if you experience heartburn and acid reflux frequently.

21. Skim milk-Who says that you cannot drink milk if you have bouts of GERD attack? Skimmed milk is ideal if you have severe GERD attack, especially if it is accompanied with pain in the breastbone area. This is very effective if you have just eaten spicy and fatty foods. To neutralize the acidity in the stomach, drink small quantities of skimmed milk every two hours in a day.

22. Probiotics-They are good bacteria that help maintain the pH balance of the gastrointestinal tract to discourage the H. pylori infection. Acidophilus are friendly microorganisms that are found in probiotics. It has the ability to remove the bad bacteria that cause sores and inflammation in the intestine.

Although there are proven and tested natural treatments for acid reflux, heartburn and GERD, sufferers should check with their doctor. The market is flooded with various herbal supplements that promise 100% effectiveness in treating these ailments, but some of them might interact with other medications that patients are taking for their existing ailments.

Chapter 5: Foods That Cause Heartburn

Food is important to keep the body and mind healthy. It is prepared using different methods of cooking so that it is pleasing to taste and smell. Various menus are introduced in restaurants to please their customers' discriminating taste. Spices, artificial sweeteners and food additives are frequently used in cooking to enhance their taste and aroma. Delectable dishes can be harmful if they are added with ingredients that can trigger heartburn.

Take a look at the list:

1. Peppermint-There is a misconception regarding the health benefits of peppermint. Although it can relieve irritable bowel syndrome and indigestion, it is not good for people who have acid reflux and GERD. Peppermint is a heartburn food because of its ability to open the sphincter muscles after eating, causing the stomach acid to move up into the esophageal lining.

2. Spicy foods-Indian and Mexican cuisines are hot and spicy that can trigger acid reflux. Avoid eating foods that are laden with chili and pepper if you have heartburn. If you really love hot and spicy foods, you may eat less, but keep a journal to record if eating a milder version can also increase the

symptoms. Examples of spicy foods are onions, garlic, and pepper.

3. Fatty foods-Fats should be avoided if you have stomach upset, hyperacidity, gastritis and heartburn as they can delay the emptying of the stomach that may cause the esophageal sphincter to open instead of closing after eating. If fatty foods cannot be avoided, take them earlier when the stomach is not full. When cooking, use a minimal amount of oil, enough to fry or sauté the food. Examples are onion rings, French fries, butter, cheese, whole milk, sour cream, meat products and cold cuts, lard, potato chips, desserts and snacks that are laden with mayonnaise, gravies, and creamy sauces.

4. Alcoholic beverages-Acid reflux is triggered if you drink alcoholic drinks such as beer, tequila, wine and champagne at dinner. If you cannot do away with alcohol, do not drink if you have a large meal or with an empty stomach as it opens the esophageal sphincter instead of closing it.

5. Citrus and tomatoes-Vegetables and fruits are great sources of vitamins, minerals and dietary fiber. Some of them can trigger or worsen the symptoms of acid reflux because they are acidic. If you have acid reflux and heartburn, avoid eating tomatoes, pineapples, limes, lemons, grapefruit and oranges. Also included are foods that are cooked with tomato paste, catsup and tomato sauce.

6. Chocolate-Eating dark chocolate is good for the heart, but chocolates can relax the lower

esophageal sphincter because it has methylxanthine. Methylxanthine is used to treat respiratory illness as it can relax the lungs' airways and soften the mucus.

Eating habits and acid reflux:

Have you noticed that while you are enjoying delectable dishes at parties, your stomach starts to rumble and you feel that burning pain below the chest area? Then that sour tasting fluid starts to flow back up into your throat.

The main culprit of this condition is the variety of foods served by the host, often is a mixture of spicy and fatty along with alcoholic drinks. Acid reflux is most common during holidays as sumptuous foods are prepared to celebrate the occasion, aside from gaining weight.

If eating these foods is unavoidable, make it a point to eat a small portion of each kind. Put aside the peppermint, nuts and spices in a saucer and be picky with the foods served. Do not ask for a second serving to play safe. Ask for water instead of alcoholic beverages and soda.

Chapter 6: Surgical Options For Acid Reflux

Acid reflux may graduate into gastroesophageal reflux disease (GERD) if it becomes frequent and occurs at least twice a week. It becomes a severe case of GERD if it does not respond to medical treatment, lifestyle and diet changes. In this case, a medical specialist will recommend surgical options to treat this medical condition.

Why is there a need for surgery?

A surgical procedure to treat gastroesophageal reflux disease, which is an advance form of acid reflux, is recommended by medical specialists if the GERD progresses and develops into complications in the esophagus such as esophagitis, bleeding of the esophagus and cancer. Surgery is an option if:

- If the symptoms of heartburn do not go away.
- If medications are ineffective.
- If non-surgical treatment is ineffective.
- Inflammation occurs in the esophagus (esophagitis)
- If there is an ulcer in the esophagus
- If there is bleeding in the esophagus
- If there is a stricture or narrowing of the esophagus.
- If Barrett's esophagus is developed.
- The symptoms are caused by stomach acid reflux.

- If you are taking medications that have contraindications with GERD medications.
- If it is caused by a hiatal hernia

A surgical procedure is the last recourse if GERD is unresponsive of the medical and homeopathic treatments. It is advisable that sufferers should undergo a physical examination to determine if there is a guarantee that the operation can address the condition. The success of the surgery will depend on the age and the overall health of the patient. Physical exams and tests include endoscopy, pH monitoring, esophageal motility study, and esophageal manometry.

Types of Surgical Procedures:

Fundoplication is the main type of surgery for acid reflux and GERD. The medical practitioner will make an incision in the stomach and the patient is given general anesthesia to prevent pain. For open surgery, the incision should be large and the doctor will operate directly using the hands.

While in the laparoscopic fundoplication, the incisions are small and the doctor operates on the patient from the outside using an instrument and will do the procedure from the outside and insert the tool into the stomach. The patient is also given a general anesthesia before the operation.

In both types of fundoplication, the surgeon will sew the incision after wrapping the top of the stomach that is close to the lower portion of the esophagus. This is to make sure that the stomach acid will stop moving up into the esophagus and allow it to heal.

Fundoplication surgery can be performed in either way, by cutting an incision in the stomach or in the chest area. Overweight patients and those with a short esophagus can benefit from the fundoplication using the chest approach.

Although laparoscopic anti-reflux surgery has many benefits, it may not be appropriate for some patients. Obtain a thorough medical evaluation by a surgeon qualified in laparoscopic anti-reflux surgery in consultation with your primary care physician or a gastroenterologist to find out if the technique is appropriate for you.

Preparation before the Surgery:

The surgeon will perform a thorough physical examination of the patient to find out the potential risks during and after the operation. The patient is asked to submit a written consent to the doctor. Submit the following requirements:

- Medical evaluation
- Chest X-ray result
- Complete blood count (CBC)
- ECG result

Preparation the day before the operation:

- Empty your bowel to have clean intestines.

- Drink only clear liquids instead of carbonated, alcoholic and powdered drinks.
- Take a shower before the operation.
- No food or drinks after midnight before the operation.
- Take only medications that are allowed by your doctor with a sip of water.
- Stop taking Vitamin E, blood thinning, anti-inflammatory and aspirin medications days or one week before the operation.
- Do not take food supplements or diet food.
- Stop smoking
- Arrange for a caregiver and domestic assistance in advance.

During the Day of Surgery:

There are many things that you need to do before the surgery to prepare you mentally and physically as there are risks involved in both open surgery and laparoscopic anti-reflux operation. However, even if there is an assurance of successful operation, complications are inevitable, which might require a second surgery.

Here's what you can do:

1. You have to wake up early to be in the hospital hours before the operation to prevent stress due to last minute preparation.

2. The nurse will place a needle in your vein to administer medication during the surgical procedure.

3. You will be given a general anesthesia to sedate you for a couple of hours.

4. After the operation, you will be transferred to the recovery room until the anesthesia has expired.

5. Depending on the type of surgery, you are advised to stay in the hospital for several days until you are strong enough to move alone.

What Happens After the Surgery?

We all know that there are two methods of fundoplication surgery to treat acid reflux and GERD. Here are things that patients should know after the surgery:

1. Open surgery-Since the incision is large, the patient will stay in the hospital for a couple of days. To avoid relapse, the patient is advised to have complete rest for four weeks to one month and a half before they can go back to their normal routine.

2. Laparoscopic fundoplication-The patient can go home after two to three days of hospital confinement. It is less painful after the procedure because the incision is small and will heal faster than the open surgery. The patient can go back to work after two to three weeks. Skilled workers should consult their physician for advice.

Surgery is not recommended for older patients, particularly for those patients who have chronic ailments. If your peristalsis or muscle movement in the esophagus is weak, surgery is not recommended because the operation may worsen the condition such as difficulty in swallowing food. If surgery is the only solution to treat GERD, partial fundoplication surgery is recommended instead of laparoscopic fundoplication which can put the patient at risk of complications that might be life threatening.

Chapter 7: Acid Reflux Postoperative Care

After the surgical procedure, the patient can expect some symptoms after the anesthesia is gone. Pain and bleeding in the abdomen are caused by the incision, including the pain inside the abdomen and esophagus where the actual operation takes place.

For patients who have laparoscopic surgery, they will notice that the symptoms of GERD have improved and the healing is faster than the open surgery. While patients who have open surgery will notice that the healing will last for a month or more. This is because of the difference in their incisions.

Some patients with esophagitis, which stemmed from simple acid reflux, may notice that the symptoms resurrect and they have to consult their doctor or might need another surgical procedure to completely remove the condition. In some patients, it is expected that symptoms may recur and in rare cases, they will experience some complications.

What are complications after surgery?

- Recurrence of heartburn
- Difficulty in swallowing food caused by overly tightened stomach wrap.

- The esophageal sphincter does not have support after the esophagus slipped out of the stomach wrap.
- Bloating because of excess gas in the stomach.
- Flatulence and colic
- Infection
- Bleeding
- Effects of anesthesia such as nausea and vomiting.

Note that fundoplication surgery is permanent. In most cases, relieving the symptoms associated with the complications of surgery is next to impossible despite another surgical procedure. Although acid reflux and GERD are not dangerous conditions, the symptoms can be irritating to the person.

Prevention is important to avoid taking the risk of complications after surgery and taking medications that may damage the kidney and the liver. Some patients are lucky to have a successful operation and this means an end in taking bitter tasting and costly medications.

Post-Operative Guidelines after Surgery:

There are many things that you must consider before you decide for an anti-reflux surgery, if this is the only way to solve your health issue. Aside from the professional fee, hospital bill and medication, you need to hire a caregiver or domestic assistant to help you while recuperating. Take a look at the following things:

Physical activity:

Complications and relapse are expected after surgical procedures for anti-reflux. The only way to prevent them is to avoid straining which will take a month to six weeks until the wound is totally healed. But this does not mean that the patient has to stop moving because inactivity can weaken the mind and the body.

Light activities such as walking or slow dancing are encouraged to stretch the muscles and strengthen the bones. Most of the time complications can happen to patients who are physically inactive.

Going back to work:

Patients may ask their doctor if they can go back to work days after their operation. Skilled workers should see to it that their operation is totally healed before going back to work. Office workers can go back to work even before their return checkup as their work cannot affect their condition.

Managing Pain:

Pain is often felt by patients after their anti-reflux surgery. The pain is caused by the incision which can be medicated with painkillers that will be taken every eight hours and to be taken with a full stomach until the pain subsides within a few days. Stop taking painkillers if the pain is tolerable. If there is pain aside from the abdomen and at the breastbone area such as shoulders, chest, back and throat, seek medical attention immediately.

Managing bowel movement:

It is normal for patients who had anti-reflux surgery to have constipation as the anesthesia and painkillers can affect the consistency of their bowel. You can take medications to loosen bowel movement that you can buy without a doctor's prescription.

To have a regular bowel movement after surgery, increase your fluid intake by drinking lots of water and fruit juices. Bloating, gas pain and stomach upset are often felt by patients after surgery because of their habit of engulfing air instead of burping. You can take anti-gas medications to relieve gas pain.

What to eat after surgery?

Patients are given a liquid diet while the esophagus and the stomach are adjusting to the operation. After a few days, the patient will have a soft diet, which is usually a small bowl of porridge or oats. Hard food should be avoided within three to six weeks because swallowing can be difficult.

As usual, do not drink soda and sugary foods. Little by little, as soon as you go home, you can try eating vegetables and fruits that are mashed to have proper digestion. Eat a small bite when eating and have a glass of water to wash down the food.

Tell your caregiver to follow the diet guide by posting a note in your kitchen. You will notice a big difference in your eating habit as your stomach can feel full easily unlike before the surgery. Keep a journal to record the food you eat until your first post-operative checkup. Some patients may vomit during mealtime. If vomiting is frequent, call your doctor for advice.

Caring the wound:

Incisions can be painful and may leave scars if you do not know how to care of the wound. Try to remove the plaster slowly but let the steri- strips stay on the skin to close the wounds and to minimize scarring. The steri-strips are durable and they can stay in the skin for a week or two. Do not cover the wound to allow circulation of air. Avoid scratching the wound when it starts to dry up by cutting your fingernails at least twice a week. If the incision becomes inflamed, call your   doctor   for   advice.

Chapter 8: Alternative Medicine For Acid Reflux

Surgery, lifestyle changes, and medications have been tried by sufferers to minimize the symptoms of acid reflux and gastroesophageal reflux disease, but to no avail. If you are getting frustrated on how to combat reflux, you can still lessen the discomfort and live normally by trying to apply alternative medicine. There is no harm if you try the alternative medicine such as acupuncture, massage therapy, relaxation techniques and hypnosis to prevent and treat acid reflux.

Acupuncture and Acid Reflux:

Acupuncture has become a popular alternative in treating various ailments, including heartburn, GERD and acid reflux. Acupuncturists use small needles to cure an illness by rebalancing the energy flow. This ancient medicine was popularized by the Chinese people for thousands of years now.

Today, the popularity of acupuncture has gained worldwide acceptance for more than three decades. It has reached the Western world and more Americans welcome acupuncture medicine to relieve pain. Acupuncture has advanced by using electro acupuncture machine. It is believed to stimulate the energy points of the body to cure the symptoms of an illness.

For the treatment of acid reflux, it relaxes the lower esophageal sphincter so that the stomach acid will not move up into the esophagus, thus minimizing irritation and bleeding.

If you wish to have an acupuncture treatment, make sure it that it will be administered by a licensed practitioner. Consult your physician before referring your condition to an acupuncturist if you have hiatal hernia, pregnant or taking other medications. The cost of acupuncture medicine may depend on the severity of your problem because you will be advised to come back for another session or more. Look for an acupuncture professional that accepts insurance plans.

Relaxation Techniques and Acid Reflux:

Are you wondering why you have acid reflux even if you are eating and avoiding foods that can trigger this condition? You do not smoke and you have an ideal weight for your height and age. Have you observed that when you are stressed, you notice that the symptoms of acid reflux recur? Stress can trigger the acid to back up into the esophagus.

This is based on a survey of 2,000 participants in 1999. It was reported that stressful situations in the home, work and travel can increase the risk of reflux disease. This is perhaps the reason why you complain of stomach upset and heartburn when you are so busy attending the needs of your family, stretching the budget and facing insurmountable problems.

Different studies and surveys have attested the connection between stress and acid reflux symptoms. Both surveys conducted by the Gallup Poll in 1993 and 1988 showed that stress is a contributor of heartburn and acid reflux.

Life events such as sickness and death in the family, wedding, divorce and business travel can aggravate the symptoms of stomach upset, gastritis, irritable bowel syndrome and acid reflux.

It is believed by scientists that the more individuals are stressed, the more that their lower esophageal sphincter is not relaxed; causing the stomach acid to flow back into the esophagus and in severe case can lead to heartburn and GERD.

Tips on how to relax:

1. Get enough sleep-Sleep can relax your mind. Do not bring your problems into your room.
2. Be physically active by indulging in physical exercises to free your mind from stressful environments. Exercise can make you feel better, younger and energetic because it loosens tight muscles and release your hormones.
3. Soothe your mind by listening to music. There are a variety of music genres that you can opt for. The most ideal is smooth jazz and relaxing music.

4. Learn a hobby-You can try doing things that you used to do when you were younger, such as painting, crocheting and knitting. There are many DIY tips about home improvement that makes your mind busy and an attractive home.

5. Practice the art of saying no-Try to turn down an invitation that is boring and less interesting. Prioritize activities that make you happy and feel good.

6. Smile and laugh-Learn to smile at people and laugh at your own mistakes instead of putting the blame on others. Watch a hilarious movie to make you laugh instead of horror and action that will only aggravate your stress.

7. Have a massage-Massage can relax your tensed muscles and mind. The relaxing music played while enjoying a massage, have calming effects on your mind.

8. Be picky with foods-People who are stressed are more likely to eat sugary and irritating foods that can trigger the symptoms of acid reflux. Instead of eating them, try to munch raw vegetables and fruits to keep your mouth busy and the mind free from worries.

9. Meditation and yoga-These are exercises that condition your mind to relax and remove the negative chi or energy that make you sick.

10. Walk with your dog-Make it a habit to walk in the morning with your furry friend. Pets can relieve your

stress. Try talking to them and teach them new tricks.

53

Chapter 9: Anti-Reflux Diet Guide

Symptoms of GERD and acid reflux can be prevented if sufferers change their lifestyle by avoiding foods that can trigger the condition. The lower esophageal sphincter (LES) acts as a valve so that food ingested into the stomach will not move backward into the esophagus. When there is an abnormality in the LES it does not close, causing the acid to move up into the esophagus. The esophageal lining gets irritated and inflamed if the reflux happens frequently in a week. Diet and proper nutrition are necessary for sufferers and those who have a surgical procedure done.

Tips on eliminating acid reflux with diet:

It was mentioned in the earlier part of this book that certain foods may trigger acid reflux such as fatty foods, hot and spicy foods and alcoholic beverages. But triggers may differ from case to case basis. It is important that sufferers should monitor their triggers by keeping a journal to avoid heartburn or acid reflux. Here are the steps to follow:

- Take note what food have you taken.
- Write the time, day and how often do you eat a certain food.
- Write down the symptoms after taking the food.
- Keep an update from time to time.
- Analyze the journal.
- Show it to your doctor.

Menu Planning:

GERD, heartburn and acid reflux have almost the same symptoms, yet treating them with lifestyle and diet changes can help a lot. There are foods that can lessen the symptoms and they are proven effective in some individuals. Before trying these foods, make sure to consult your doctor and ask for recommendations because its efficacy might differ from one person to another, especially if they have an existing ailment other than gastroesophageal reflux disease. Prepare meals that are high in fiber, but low in acid and fat.

Take a run down at the following recipes:

1. Banana Oat Ginger Smoothie

Ingredients:

- ½ cup crushed ice
- 2 cups oats
- 2 ripe Cavendish bananas
- 1 cup yogurt
- ½ teaspoon fresh ginger, grated
- 2 tablespoon honey

Procedure:

- In a blender, add the ice, oats, yogurt, bananas and ginger.
- Blend well until the mixture is smooth.
- Add the honey. Serve cold.

2. Banana Apple Aloe Vera Smoothie

Ingredients:

- 2 ripe Cavendish bananas
- 1 apple cored and cut in half
- 5 tablespoons aloe vera
- 2 cups crushed ice
- 1 teaspoon grated orange peel
- 1 teaspoon honey

Procedure:

- In a blender, add the ice, bananas, apple, aloe vera, orange peel.
- Blend the mixture until smooth.
- Add the honey and stir the mixture. Serve cold.

3. Oatmeal Cantaloupe Apple Refrigerator Delight

Ingredients:

- 1 ½ cup instant oatmeal
- 1 cup milk
- 2 tablespoons raisins
- 1 cup sliced cantaloupe, cored
- 1 apple, cored and diced
- 2 teaspoons honey
- Pinch of salt

Directions:

- Mix the instant oatmeal, milk, raisins, honey and salt in a large bowl
- Chill overnight or three hours before serving.
- Adjust the taste by adding milk if the mixture is too thick. Ready to serve.

4. Banana Cornmeal Soup

Ingredients:

- 2 cups cornmeal
- 3 ripe Cavendish bananas
- 1 teaspoon vanilla extract
- 1 teaspoon lime zest
- 2 tablespoons honey
- 2 ½ cups whole milk
- Pinch of salt

Directions:

- Heat the whole milk in slow fire.
- Add the cornmeal and stir to avoid curdling.
- Add the bananas, vanilla extract, lime zest, salt and honey.
- Serve warm.

5. Carrot Turnip Salad

Ingredients:

- ½ pound grated carrots
- ½ pound grated turnips
- 2 tablespoons raisins
- 2 tablespoons olive oil
- 2 tablespoons lime juice
- 2 tablespoons honey
- 1 teaspoon dried oregano
- Pinch of salt

Directions:

- In a large mixing bowl, toss the lime juice, honey, olive oil, dried oregano and salt. Chill in the refrigerator for 20 minutes.
- Pour the mixture over the vegetables and toss.
- Adjust the taste by adding salt if needed.
- Serve cold.

6. Mung Bean with Milk Soup:

Ingredients:

- 1 cup mung beans
- 2 cups whole milk
- 1 cup water
- 1 teaspoon nonfat sour cream
- Pinch of salt
- 2 teaspoons sugar

Procedure:

- Soak the mung beans overnight.
- The following morning rinse the mung beans, removing the outer skin.
- Boil the mung beans in water for 25 to 30 minutes. Stir occasionally to avoid burning.
- When the mixture is consistent, add the milk, and stir to avoid curdling.
- Season with sugar and a pinch of salt.
- Add the nonfat sour cream before serving.

These are samples recipes to prevent acid reflux and for postoperative care. You can combine different fruits and vegetables to have a variation. Just study the procedure how they are prepared. You can make salads, soups and smoothies for your meals and snacks. You can also include cereal, fish, nonfat or low fat dairy products, lean meat, parsley, apples, brown rice, and shredded chicken. For salads, include olive oil, balsamic vinaigrette and toasted walnuts.

Conclusion

Acid reflux, though not dangerous, might lead to other illness if the symptoms occur several times a week. Acid reflux is accompanied with backing up of the acid that tastes bitter and sour right into the esophagus. The symptoms may last for more than an hour, causing discomfort and annoyance to the sufferer.

Most sufferers are disappointed with the result of their treatment as the symptoms continue to haunt them, especially at night. Acid reflux is one of the most popular searches online as more and more people are affected by this condition. In lieu of this concern, this book is conceptualized to help sufferers prevent and cure their reflux disease before surgery is performed as the last recourse.

Part 2

Chapter 1 - What is Acid Reflux?

Most people would assume it's the burning sensation you get in your chest that can be anywhere from a mild annoyance to a debilitating pain so intense all you can do is squeeze yourself tightly and moan. When in fact, that's only part of it.

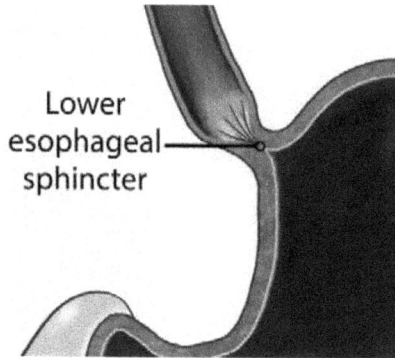

Lower esophageal sphincter

There is an opening at the top of the stomach called the esophageal sphincter. This is the part of the stomach which opens to allow entering the stomach but preventing the digestive acids from entering the esophagus. However, when you suffer from reflux, the LES does not shut completely, allowing some of the acids to backup into the esophagus.

This is commonly known as Acid Reflux Disease, but it is also classified as Gastroesophageal Reflux Disease. Most people who suffer from acid reflux also suffer from hiatal hernia. A hiatal hernia is when the upper stomach and LES shift above the diaphragm. One of the symptoms of hiatal hernia is the feeling of something getting "stuck" in your throat.

Now that we know what it is, we need to get to the root causes of how it comes to be and what can trigger it.

• Not eating for a long period of time. This is not a common cause, but it does happen. The best way to prevent reflux due to this is to eat small meals and snacks through the day.

• Stress is a factor. When you are in a high stress situation or in a situation that prolongs stress, it tends to wear down the weakest system in the body. If you have always had a weak digestive system, then it can turn into either an intestinal illness or acid reflux.

• Eating large portion meals can cause reflux. It's better to make portion sizes which are nutritionally balanced. At first glance, the portions will look small, but then you put it all together for a meal, it can be a lot of food.

• Lying down immediately after eating can also contribute to reflux. It generally takes a minimum of three hours to digest most of the food you eat at mealtime. Lying down can slow the digestive process, and if your LES does not close completely, the acid can leak into the esophagus.

• Obesity or being overweight can contribute to reflux. Being overweight puts pressure on the body, and the more fat you have on your body, the more it compresses your internal organs, making them work harder. It works the same with your stomach.

• Eating rich foods in meal and then lying down, even bending over can make the acid leak into the esophagus. Eating rich foods, like pasts dishes or other heavy foods can make you feel tired. This is due to your body rerouting the energy to help with digestion. Eat smaller portions of the rich foods to avoid the food coma and you should be okay.

• Eating is to close to bedtime. This one is related to lying down shortly after eating. It is always recommended that the last meal of the day should be eaten no later than six in the evening. This will give your digestive system time to work its magic.

• Eating foods high in citric acid, tomatoes, garlic, onions, even spicy and fatty foods can trigger it. Some can't eat minty foods. Your food triggers may vary from someone else. In order to find your triggers, make a journal of the foods you eat that give you reflux. In the case of orange juice, try the juice fresh, not from concentrate to see if that helps prevent a flare-up. The same goes for drinks like alcohol and so forth.

• Being a smoker can cause flare-ups as well.

• If you are pregnant, there is a chance you may have instances of reflux.

● Certain medications can cause it, too (especially, non-steroidal anti-inflammatory drugs or antibiotics).

- You may also have food allergy and don't know about it. Reflux can be a manifestation of food allergy, then it would be better to make an analysis IgG4 testing food intolerance and then exclude allergens (by the way it can help you not only fight a reflux, but improve your health. maybe you don't know about your individual intolerance to some healthy products because sometimes it doesn't have immediate reactions)

- Peptic ulcer disease and Gastritis (both of them can be caused by some factors such as Helicobacter Pylori or Inherited factors)

These are the most common reasons.

There is some advice on how to help yourself, but don't forget if you want to fight a disease you must find a reason. So it's better to start from a medical examination.

A note on prescriptions for reflux

If you are prescribed medications for acid reflux, you may find that running out will make the condition worse. This is due to the medicine's design of shutting off some of the valves that produce the acid. When the medication leaves your system, the valves will re-activate, causing a worse episode than before you started taking it. Your body is overcompensating. I am not telling you stop taking the medication, just advising you that this may be a cause of how it seems to be worse when you run out.

Serious Signs

Regular reflux can be managed by diet and some medications, but there are instances where you may need to take more drastic steps to keep your reflux regulated. Here are some symptoms to look out for:

• Constant bloating no matter what you eat. To give your doctor a better idea of the severity, mark down when you experience bloating.

• If your stools are bloody and/or black or if you have blood in your vomit. See a physician immediately.

• Constant burping. This may be related to bloating.

• Unrelenting hiccups.

• When your esophagus narrows and gives you a feeling of food being stuck.

• If you start losing weight for no reason, you need to contact your physician.

• If you have a constant sore throat, you wheeze, have a dry cough or are constantly hoarse.

• Being constantly nauseated.

Chapter 2 - The Digestive System

We are going to go a little deeper into how the gastrointestinal tract and how to maintain a balance to prevent reflux and other digestive problems.

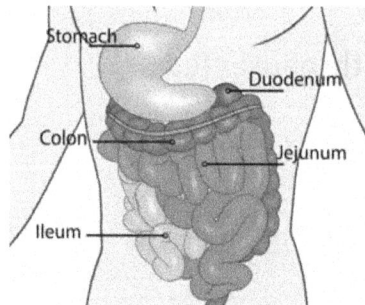

The Stomach

This is the first stop any food and drink taken in makes before continuing its journey. It is met with stomach acids and enzymes to break down the food and drink:

Pepsin, renni, hydrochloric acid, and mucus are the main acids and enzymes which make digestion happen in the stomach. Pepsin converts protein to make the substance easily absorbed. The hydrochloric acid helps the pepsin do the conversion. The rennin helps the stomach breakdown milk proteins. Mucus coats the lining of the stomach to protect the lining from the gastric juices. Hormones and certain chemical substances tend to stimulate acid and enzyme secretion. Only 10 percent of the digestive process is in the stomach.

The Small Intestine and Duodenum

As the substances in stomach get digested, they make their way to the small intestine. The rest of the digestion happens here, in the small intestine. It is here where the absorption of food and nutrients occurs. This is where the bulk of the enzymes and bile acids break down the foods to get them ready for adsorption. Once absorbed, the nutrients are conveyed to the blood stream and other parts of the body.

Colon

This is also known as the large intestine. The rest of the food is pushed here to travel to the anus.

PH Balance of the Digestive System

As scientists test certain substances for pH, your body has to maintain a pH balance in order to function properly and prevent reflux and other digestive problems. In the digestive system, your saliva is in the 6.5 to 7.5 range, which makes it balanced. In the upper stomach, the acidity dips to 4.0 to start the breakdown of food, and then continues to become more acidic at 1.0 in the lower part of the stomach. The small intestine ranges from 4.0 to 7.0, which matches the colon.

Balancing Your Body's pH

In order to balance your body's pH, you need to get a reading of what your body's pH is before you make the decision of changing your body chemistry. You do this by purchasing a pH test and administering it when you urinate for the first time before you eat or drink anything. That is when you can get the most accurate reading. If your body registers in the highly acidic range, you need to look for foods that are alkaline in nature to bring it back into balance. Here is a short list of alkaline foods.

Alkaline foods

7.0-Neutral

- Butter

- Fresh cream with no salt

- Raw milk

- Most tap water (test yours to make sure)

8.0

- Apples

- Almonds

- Avocados

- Tomatoes

- Fresh corn

- Mushrooms

- Turnips

- Olives

- Soybeans

- Bell peppers

- Radishes

- Rhubarb

- Pineapple

- Cherries

- Millet

- Wild rice

- Strawberries

- Apricots

- Cantaloupe

- Honeydew

- Peaches

- Oranges

- Grapefruit

- Bananas

9.0

- Olive oil

- Herbal tea

- Sprouted grains

- Green tea

- Borage oil

- Raw zucchini

- Papayas

- Figs

- Blueberries

- Raw peas

- Most lettuce

- Raw eggplant

- Raw green beans

- Beets

- Greens

- Alfalfa sprouts

- Pears

- Mangoes

- Melons

- Kiwi

- Dates

- Sweet potato

- Tangerines

- Grapes

10.0

- Raw spinach

- Collards

- Artichokes

- Red cabbage

- Carrots

- Raw celery

- Cauliflower

- Raw broccoli

- Potato skins

- Asparagus

- Lemons

- Alfalfa grass

- Brussels sprouts

- Cucumbers

- Seaweed

- Onions

- Limes

Things to take note

On your road to bringing you body back into balance, there are a few things to keep in mind:

● To counteract 1 part of acidity in the body, you need to intake 20 parts of foods and liquids that are alkaline in nature.

● Some of the foods on the alkaline chart will become acidic when cooked.

● The best way to intake some of the foods on the chart is raw, such as in salads.

Chapter 3 - Adjusting Your Diet

I know I briefly covered this in the previous chapter, but it needs to expand a bit. There are foods which will trigger reflux, and we will discuss some of those here. I will also cover some foods that can help when an attack comes on.

Foods to avoid

High-acid foods

Most people think oranges and tomatoes, and they would be correct, but there are more foods that are acidic to consider. Any food that is high in citric acid or ascorbic acid (Vitamin C) can also trigger reflux. Some people will shy away from drinking orange juice because of the pain it induces, but most of the juice is concentrated. There are a couple of companies that do not make orange juice concentrated. The "Simply" brand is one. There are people I know that can drink the juices from that company, in small servings, and not have reflux.

Spicy foods
Everyone loves a good chili and others a good spicy curry or soup, but the enzymes and acidic nature of the spices can trigger reflux, leaving you in agony.

Onions and Garlic

These are two foods that can vary between people. Some can eat them with no problem, others in small doses, and others not at all. There is an enzyme in both can may cause flare-ups.

Caffeine

Coffee, soft drinks, chocolate all have one thing in common. They all contain caffeine. It could be the caffeine that can spark a flare-up, and in soft drinks, it could also be the carbonation.

Mint

This can be a trigger for some and not be one for others.

Foods that help

We all hate the list of foods we have to avoid, but did you know there were foods out there that help to curve, prevent, or in some cases, stop a flare-up? Here you go.

Oatmeal

Oatmeal is filling and can also help stave off a flare-up due to its ability to absorb liquids. It can also counter acid in foods like raisins and apples.

Ginger

Used in small bits, is can help with flare-ups as well as be a treatment for reflux. I know it seems counter-productive because of its acidic nature, but it is highly recommended for many digestive problems.

Aloe Vera

The juice from this plant can help with reflux other digestive problems.

Salads/salad greens

A good salad is alkaline in nature and can neutralize many acids in the stomach.

Banana

This is a fruit that is used to balance the pH in the system, reducing acidity.

Melon

This is another alkaline fruit that counters highly acidic foods.

Fennel

Usually used for seasoning, this herb is highly recommended for treating reflux. It also makes a good snack for those who like a licorice taste.

Chicken and Turkey

Boiled, baked, grilled, or sautéed without the skin.

Fish and seafood

Baked, grilled, sautéed, but not fried. Also wild caught would be preferable to farm raised.

Roots and Cruciferous Vegetables

Broccoli, green beans and the like are all great for those who suffer from reflex.

Parsley

Often the garnish on a plate in a high-end restaurant, chewing on a sprig of this can quell a reflux flare-up.

Papaya

This fruit contains an enzyme that can break down proteins into amino acids. It can also do wonders for acid reflux.

Water

Water is a very important substance. There is some advice on how to drink: food and water preferable take separately. In the morning it's good to take one cup of warm mineral water.

Chapter 4 - Herbal Supplements

In the natural health field, there are some herbs that you can either add to your food or take in capsule form to help with heartburn/reflux. You can even make some into a tea. We will go into that here.

Agrimony

You can use this herb to help with stomach upset and to help even out functions of the gastrointestinal tract. Agrimony is super effective in treating reflux, nausea, diarrhea, and vomiting.

Fenugreek seeds

This is a seed that creates a gel. This gel acts like a sponge, soaking up any excess acid in the system. The best part about these seeds is that they can be sprinkled on food and eaten with any preparation needed.

German Chamomile

This herb has been used for centuries to help with digestive issues including reflux and other heartburn issues. It is also good for general stomach pains.

Licorice

This herb not only helps with flare-ups, but it can also help heal damage done by reflux.

Slippery Elm

The bark of this tree has gelling properties that can absorb excess acid and other fluids, too. It can also sooth irritated stomach lining.

Turmeric

This herb has been found to have many healing properties, and they are finding more every day. Some discoveries include the ability to stop flare-ups, prevent future ones, arresting inflammation, and also instant relief of gas and bloating.

Recipes

Licorice and Chamomile Tea

1 tsp German Chamomile

1 tsp Licorice Root

- Bring two cups of water to a boil
- Add the licorice
- Reduce to medium boil for 15 minutes
- Place Chamomile in the pot
- Cover pot and steep for 10 minutes
- Strain out the herbs and add honey

Reflux Syrup

1/2 Ounce Slippery Elm

1/2 Ounce German Chamomile

1/2 Ounce Fenugreek Seeds

1/2 Ounce Fennel Root

1 Quart Water

2 Ounces Glycerin or Honey

- Add the herbs to the water.
- Boil the water down to a pint
- Strain out the herbs
- Add the honey or glycerin
- Mix well and let cool
- Take one tablespoon on flare-ups

Ginger Oil

8 Ounces Olive Oil

1 Ounce Ginger root

- Place in the Ginger and oil in a tinted glass bottle
- Close with a tight lid
- Leave in a cool dry place for two weeks
- Use in cooking recipes

Fennel and Fenugreek Oil

1 Ounces of Olive Oil

3 tbsp Fenugreek seeds

2 tbsp Dried Fennel

Follow instructions above

Digestion Oil

1/2 Ounce Agrimony

1/2 Ounce German Chamomile

1/2 Ounce Dried Fennel

1/2 Ounce Tumeric

1 Quart Water

2 Ounces Glycerin or Honey

- Add the herbs to the water.
- Boil the water down to a pint
- Strain out the herbs
- Add the honey or glycerin
- Mix well and let cool
- Take one tablespoon on flare-ups

Tips and Tricks

Baking Soda Trick

1 tsp Baking Soda

1/4 Cup water

- Dissolve the backing in the water
- Drink

There is a warning to this one. It does taste horrible. So have something to chase it with when you are done. You will burp, and as you burp, you will feel better. Depending on the severity, you may to do it more than once.

Peppermint

Though some would say mint makes it worse, peppermint can help a lot of many by cooling you from the inside out.

Sleep at an angle

Sleeping flat when you feel an attack coming is never a good idea. Sleep at a 45 degree angle for some relief until your treatment kicks in.

Exercise

This one is not as easy to do during a flare up, but walking will help get gasses moving and help you alleviate a flare-up along with any other treatments.

Food Diary

Log down all the foods you eat in a day, and log down your body's reactions to the food. If you have a flare up, make sure it's the actual type of you just ate and not one of the ingredients. Sometimes it's not the main part of the dish or side item, but a simple little ingredient that did it. Look for common ingredients.

Baking Soda

If you want to make pasta with marinara, but are dreading the burn after, put a pinch of baking soda in the sauce. The pinch should not be larger than half a pea size. Any more and the sauce will taste funny. It will counteract the acid in the tomato sauce.

Herb Shops
In some herb shops or health foods stores, you will find papaya and mint tablets. These are normally chewable and work better than Tums and other antacids you can get at conventional stores. You can also find Fenugreek and fennel in capsules and by the ounce, too. These stores often sell pure Aloe Vera juice and all the herbs on the list in this chapter. Don't be afraid to ask the shop manager if there are other alternative as well.

Chapter 5 – Recipes to regulate the acidity

Here are some recipes you can try to regulate the acidity and help to regulate reflux.

Banana Nut Oatmeal

1/2 Cup Steel Cut Oats

1 1/2 Cups water

2 Medium Size Ripe bananas

1 tsp vanilla extract

1/2 tsp nutmeg

1/2 tsp cinnamon

1/8 Cup brown sugar

Pinch of salt

- Mash the bananas
- Mix the sugar, nutmeg, vanilla, and cinnamon into the bananas
- Bring the water to a boil
- Add the salt
- Stir in the banana mixture
- Let simmer for five minutes
- Bring it back to a boil and add the oats
- Simmer covered until soft, about 15 minutes

Grilled Chicken Salad

3 ounces grilled chicken, chopped

1/4 Cup raw Spinach

1/4 Cup Romaine Lettuce

1/4 cup Cucumber, peeled and chopped

1/4 Cup Baby Bella mushrooms, chopped

1/4 Cup sliced Strawberries

2 tbsp sliced Almonds

1 tbsp Olive Oil

1/2 lemon Juiced

- Mix the vegetables in a bowl
- Top with the chicken
- Drizzle the oil and lemon
- Toss once more and eat

Morning Juice

1/4 cup Zucchini

5 Strawberries

1/2 Pear

3 Sprigs of Parsley

1/2 Red Apple

Run all through a juicer and drink before your meal. It will help with digestion.

Yogurt Smoothie

1/2 cup yogurt

1 medium banana

1/4 papaya chunks

6 Strawberries

1/4 Cup Pineapple

Blend all in a blender and add ice to thicken.

Melon Salad

1/4 Cup Honeydew

1/4 Cup Cantaloupe

1/2 Cup Vanilla Yogurt

Mix together and eat as a snack or with a meal.

Even though the list of foods may seem limited, but there a lot of things you can do with the foods take keep your digestive system functioning normally. Challenge yourself by adding a food you've never tried before to your daily intake. Step out of your comfort zone. You will be surprised at the foods will like that you didn't think you would.

Chapter 6 – Stress

You can't fully address digestive problems without touching on one of the reasons our bodies are more prone to illness and disorders.

In our everyday lives, we encounter stress and stressful situations. Between paying bills, balancing budgets, balancing work with recreation, we tend to get overwhelmed. This causes stress. Here are some things you can do to reduce it.

Exercise

This can be anything from just taking a walk to joining a gym. Find a type of exercise you like, and you will be more likely to stick with it. Two highly recommended exercises are Yoga and Thai Chi.

Meditation

Mediating can be a great way to relieve stress. There are many ways to meditate, but if you would like an easy method, here is a quick guide to Fixed-Point Meditation:

• Light a candle or pick a spot on a wall to concentrate on.

• Breathe in slowly as you isolate and tighten a muscle group.

• Exhale slowly as you relax the muscle group, concentrating on the point you chose to focus on.

• Repeat the process until you have tightened and relaxed all of the muscles in your body.

Read a Book

Sometimes the best way to relieve stress is to immerse yourself in something that sparks your imagination. Reading a book does just that. A good book will keep your attention focused on the story and provide you the break you need from the everyday stresses.

Spoil Yourself

We tend to get so wrapped up in caring for others we forget to pamper ourselves. A soak in a tub, a trip to a spa for a massage or facial treatment can be great ways to pamper and spoil you.

Take Up a Hobby

Find something you like doing, like drawing, writing, or even crafting. Taking up a hobby can also take your mind of stress.

Unplug

This may be the hardest one on the list to do, but you are exposing your mind to constant stimulus when you check your social media, emails, surf the web and even text. Designate a time during the day to unplug all electronics and just do something that does not need a computer to do. A few suggestions have been listed above.

Play/Hang Out

Take time out of your day to play with your kids if you have a family or make dates to hang out with friends to talk or have fun. Either one will help you relieve stress and help you be healthy.

In this book you can find some advice how to improve your situation, but don't forget if you want to solve your problem you must find a reason. So it's better to start from a medical examination.

Medical advice

If you suffer from acid reflux it can be a signal that you have some problems in your body.

1. Check your liver and pancreas and stomach.

The process of food digestion is very complicated. There are lots of substances (such as enzymes, HCl) used in digestion process and there is a balance between them). When the balance is broken you can get some negative consequences such as reflux. So it's recommended to visit your physician. He can advise you to make Esophagogastroduodenoscopy or get some tests.

2. Check if you have food intolerance

Get IgG4 testing food intolerance?

3. Check if you have Helicobacter Pylori

Get a blood test IgG on Helicobacter Pylori.

4. Try to avoid non-steroidal anti-inflammatory drugs or antibiotics.

SOUP RECIPES

ROASTED JALAPENO SOUP

Serves: **4**

Prep Time: **10**   Minutes

Cook Time: **20**   Minutes

Total Time: 30   Minutes

INGREDIENTS

1 tablespoon olive oil
1 tablespoon roasted jalapeno
¼ red onion
½ cup all-purpose flour
¼ tsp salt
¼ tsp pepper
1 can vegetable broth
1 cup heavy cream

DIRECTIONS

1. In a saucepan heat olive oil and sauté onion until tender
2. Add remaining ingredients to the saucepan and bring to a boil

3. When all the vegetables are tender transfer to a blender and blend until smooth

4. Pour soup into bowls, garnish with parsley and serve

PARSNIP SOUP

Serves: **4**

Prep Time: **10** Minutes

Cook Time: **20** Minutes

Total Time: 30 Minutes

INGREDIENTS

1 tablespoon olive oil
1 cup parsnip
¼ red onion
½ cup all-purpose flour
¼ tsp salt
¼ tsp pepper
1 can vegetable broth
1 cup heavy cream

DIRECTIONS

1. In a saucepan heat olive oil and sauté parsnip until tender

2. Add remaining ingredients to the saucepan and bring to a boil

3. When all the vegetables are tender transfer to a blender and blend until smooth

4. Pour soup into bowls, garnish with parsley and serve

SPINACH SOUP

Serves: **4**

Prep Time: **10** Minutes

Cook Time: **20** Minutes

Total Time: 30 Minutes

INGREDIENTS

1 tablespoon olive oil
1 lb. spinach
¼ red onion
½ cup all-purpose flour
¼ tsp salt
¼ tsp pepper
1 can vegetable broth
1 cup heavy cream

DIRECTIONS

1. In a saucepan heat olive oil and sauté spinach until tender
2. Add remaining ingredients to the saucepan and bring to a boil

3. When all the vegetables are tender transfer to a blender and blend until smooth

4. Pour soup into bowls, garnish with parsley and serve

CUCUMBER SOUP

Serves: **4**

Prep Time: **10**   Minutes

Cook Time: **20**   Minutes

Total Time: 30   Minutes

INGREDIENTS

1 tablespoon olive oil
1 lb. cucumber
¼ red onion
½ cup all-purpose flour
¼ tsp salt
¼ tsp pepper
1 can vegetable broth
1 cup heavy cream

DIRECTIONS

1. In a saucepan heat olive oil and sauté onion until tender
2. Add remaining ingredients to the saucepan and bring to a boil

3. When all the vegetables are tender transfer to a blender and blend until smooth

4. Pour soup into bowls, garnish with parsley and serve

SWEETCORN SOUP

Serves: **4**

Prep Time: **10** Minutes

Cook Time: **20** Minutes

Total Time: 30   Minutes

INGREDIENTS

1 tablespoon olive oil
1 lb. sweetcorn
¼ red onion
½ cup all-purpose flour
¼ tsp salt
¼ tsp pepper
1 can vegetable broth
1 cup heavy cream

DIRECTIONS

1. In a saucepan heat olive oil and sauté onion until tender
2. Add remaining ingredients to the saucepan and bring to a boil

3. When all the vegetables are tender transfer to a blender and blend until smooth

4. Pour soup into bowls, garnish with parsley and serve

SIDE DISHES

GREEN PESTO PASTA

Serves: **2**

Prep Time: **5**   Minutes

Cook Time: **15**   Minutes

Total Time: 20   Minutes

INGREDIENTS

4 oz. spaghetti
2 cups basil leaves
2 garlic cloves
¼ cup olive oil
2 tablespoons parmesan cheese
½ tsp black pepper

DIRECTIONS

1. Bring water to a boil and add pasta
2. In a blend add parmesan cheese, basil leaves, garlic and blend
3. Add olive oil, pepper and blend again
4. Pour pesto onto pasta and serve when ready

CHICKEN AND BROCCOLI

Serves: **4**

Prep Time: **5**   Minutes

Cook Time: **10** Minutes

Total Time: 15   Minutes

INGREDIENTS

1 lb chicken thighs
1 ½ tbs sesame seeds
2 tsp garlic
1/3 cup oyster sauce
2 tbs oil

1/3 cup chicken broth
2 tsp honey
1 tsp sesame oil
2 cups broccoli florets
1 ½ tsp soy sauce
1 tsp cornstarch
Salt

Pepper

DIRECTIONS

1. Cook the broccoli in hot oil until tender
2. Add the garlic and cook 30 more seconds
3. Place the seasoned chicken in the pan and cook until browned
4. Mix the oyster sauce, honey, soy sauce, chicken broth and sesame oil together
5. Combine the cornstarch with 1 tbs of cold water
6. Pour the oyster mixture over the chicken and broccoli and cook for 30 seconds
7. Add the cornstarch, bring to a boil and cook for a minute
8. Serve topped with sesame seeds

CHICKEN AND RICE

Serves: **4**

Prep Time: **10**   Minutes

Cook Time: **20**   Minutes

Total Time: 30   Minutes

INGREDIENTS

1 cup rice
15 oz salsa
3 tsp paprika
3 tbs olive oil
1 ½ cup chicken broth
2 lb chicken thigh

DIRECTIONS

1. Cut the chicken and toss with the paprika
2. Cook in hot oil until browned
3. Add the rice and mix well, cooking 1 more minute to toast the rice
4. Add the broth and salsa and stir

5. Bring to a simmer, then cover and cook for 20 minutes
6. Serve immediately

EASY TACOS

Serves: **8**

Prep Time: **10**   Minutes

Cook Time: **20**   Minutes

Total Time: 30   Minutes

INGREDIENTS

Tortilla shells
3 bell peppers
2 tbs olive oil
2 cups green lentils
1 onion

3 cloves garlic
3 cups mushrooms
1 package taco seasoning
2 tsp paprika
1 cup water
Parsley

DIRECTIONS

1. Sauté the peppers in hot oil until soft

2. Add the onions and garlic and cook until soft
3. Add the mushrooms, lentils, paprika and taco seasoning and stir until the mushrooms release some juice
4. Add the water slowly to create a sauce
5. Reduce the heat and cook for 15 minutes
6. Add the bell peppers and combine
7. Place the mixture onto each taco shell
8. Serve immediately

BBQ CHICKEN

Serves: *4*

Prep Time: *10*   Minutes

Cook Time: *5*   Hours

Total Time: 40   Minutes

INGREDIENTS

1/3 cup chicken broth
1 cup BBQ sauce
1 ½ lbs chicken breasts

DIRECTIONS

1. Place the ingredients in a crockpot and cook on low for 5 hours

2. Break the meat to shred

3. Serve over a bun

TUNA MELTS

Serves: **2**

Prep Time: **5**   Minutes

Cook Time: **5**   Minutes

Total Time: 10   Minutes

INGREDIENTS

6 oz tuna

3 tbs onion
¼ tsp salt
¼ tsp black pepper
1 avocado

3 tbs Greek yogurt
3 oz cheese
2 tomatoes

DIRECTIONS

1. Mix together onion, tuna, diced avocado, Greek yogurt, salt, and pepper
2. Place tomato slices on a baking sheet on a wire rack
3. To each slice with tuna mixture, then top with cheese

4. Broil until cheese is melted

CAPRESE SALAD

Serves: **2**

Prep Time: **5**   Minutes

Cook Time: **5**   Minutes

Total Time: 10   Minutes

INGREDIENTS

3 cups tomatoes
2 oz. mozzarella cheese
2 tablespoons basil
1 tablespoon olive oil

DIRECTIONS

1. In a bowl combine all ingredients together and mix well
2. Serve with dressing

BUTTERNUT SQUASH SALAD

Serves: **2**

Prep Time: **5**   Minutes

Cook Time: **5**   Minutes

Total Time: 10   Minutes

INGREDIENTS

3 cups butternut squash
1 cup cooked couscous
2 cups kale leaves
2 tablespoons cranberries
2 oz. goat cheese
1 cup salad dressing

DIRECTIONS

1. In a bowl combine all ingredients together and mix
    well
2. Serve with dressing

TURKEY SALAD

Serves: **2**

Prep Time: **5**   Minutes

Cook Time: **5**   Minutes

Total Time: 10   Minutes

INGREDIENTS

2 tablespoons lemon juice
2 tablespoons roasted garlic
2 tablespoons olive oil
1 tablespoon honey
2 cups cooked turkey breast
1 cup berries
1 cup green onions

DIRECTIONS

1. In a bowl combine all ingredients together and mix well
2. Serve with dressing

CANTALOUPE SALAD

Serves: **2**

Prep Time: **5** Minutes

Cook Time: **5** Minutes

Total Time: 10 Minutes

INGREDIENTS

2 cups watermelon
1 cup cantaloupe
1 tablespoon honey
1 tablespoon mint
1 tsp basil leaves
½ cup feta cheese

DIRECTIONS

1. In a bowl combine all ingredients together and mix well
2. Serve with dressing

CORN SALAD

Serves: **2**

Prep Time: **5**   Minutes

Cook Time: **5**   Minutes

Total Time: 10   Minutes

INGREDIENTS

1 cup corn
1 cup cucumber
1 cup tomatoes
¼ cup avocado
1 tablespoon lime juice
½ cup Greek yogurt
1 cup salad dressing

DIRECTIONS

1. In a bowl combine all ingredients together and mix well
2. Serve with dressing

SALMON EGG SALAD

Serves: **2**

Prep Time: **5**   Minutes

Cook Time: **5**   Minutes

Total Time: 10   Minutes

INGREDIENTS

2 hard boiled eggs
¼ cup red onion
2 tablespoons capers
1 tablespoon lime juice
3 oz. smoked salmon
1 tablespoon olive oil

DIRECTIONS

1. In a bowl combine all ingredients together and mix
   well
2. Serve with dressing

QUINOA SALAD

Serves: **2**

Prep Time: **5**   Minutes

Cook Time: **5**   Minutes

Total Time: 10   Minutes

INGREDIENTS

1 cup cooked quinoa
1 tablespoon olive oil
1 tablespoon mustard
2 tablespoons lemon juice
1 cucumber
½ red onion
½ cup almonds
1 tablespoon mint

DIRECTIONS

1. In a bowl combine all ingredients together and mix well
2. Serve with dressing

GREEK SALAD

Serves: **2**

Prep Time: **5**   Minutes

Cook Time: **5**   Minutes

Total Time: 10   Minutes

INGREDIENTS

1 cup cucumber
¼ cup tomatoes
¼ cup red onion
¼ cup avocado
¼ cup feta cheese
1 tablespoon olives
¼ pecans

1 tablespoon vinegar
1 tsp olive oil

DIRECTIONS

1. In a bowl combine all ingredients together and mix
    well
2. Serve with dressing

AVOCADO SALAD

Serves: **2**

Prep Time: **5** Minutes

Cook Time: **5** Minutes

Total Time: 10 Minutes

INGREDIENTS

1 cup corn
1 cup tomatoes
1 cup cucumber
½ cup avocado
½ cup edamame
1 cup salad dressing

DIRECTIONS

1. In a bowl combine all ingredients together and mix well
2. Serve with dressing

ENDIVE FRITATTA

Serves: **2**

Prep Time: **10**   Minutes

Cook Time: **20**   Minutes

Total Time: 30   Minutes

INGREDIENTS

½ lb. endive
1 tablespoon olive oil
½ red onion
2 eggs

¼ tsp salt
2 oz. cheddar cheese
1 garlic clove
¼ tsp dill

DIRECTIONS

1. In a bowl whisk eggs with salt and cheese
2. In a frying pan heat olive oil and pour egg mixture
3. Add remaining ingredients and mix well
4. Serve when ready

BOK CHOY FRITATTA

Serves: **2**

Prep Time: **10** Minutes

Cook Time: **20** Minutes

Total Time: 30 Minutes

INGREDIENTS

½ lb. bok choy
1 tablespoon olive oil
½ red onion
¼ tsp salt
2 eggs

2 oz. cheddar cheese
1 garlic clove
¼ tsp dill

DIRECTIONS

1. In a bowl whisk eggs with salt and cheese
2. In a frying pan heat olive oil and pour egg mixture
3. Add remaining ingredients and mix well
4. Serve when ready

KALE FRITATTA

Serves: **2**

Prep Time: **10** Minutes

Cook Time: **20** Minutes

Total Time: 30 Minutes

INGREDIENTS

1 cup kale
1 tablespoon olive oil
½ red onion
¼ tsp salt
2 oz. cheddar cheese
1 garlic clove
2 eggs

¼ tsp dill

DIRECTIONS

1. In a bowl whisk eggs with salt and cheese
2. In a frying pan heat olive oil and pour egg mixture
3. Add remaining ingredients and mix well
4. Serve when ready

LEEK FRITATTA

Serves: **2**

Prep Time: **10**   Minutes

Cook Time: **20**   Minutes

Total Time: 30   Minutes

INGREDIENTS

½ cup leek
1 tablespoon olive oil
½ red onion
2 eggs

¼ tsp salt
2 oz. parmesan cheese
1 garlic clove
¼ tsp dill

DIRECTIONS

1. In a bowl whisk eggs with salt and cheese
2. In a frying pan heat olive oil and pour egg mixture
3. Add remaining ingredients and mix well

4. Serve when ready

BROCCOLI FRITATTA

Serves: **2**

Prep Time: **10** Minutes

Cook Time: **20** Minutes

Total Time: 30 Minutes

INGREDIENTS

1 cup broccoli
1 tablespoon olive oil
½ red onion
2 eggs

¼ tsp salt
2 oz. cheddar cheese
1 garlic clove
¼ tsp dill

DIRECTIONS

1. In a bowl whisk eggs with salt and cheese
2. In a frying pan heat olive oil and pour egg mixture
3. Add remaining ingredients and mix well
4. Serve when ready

LEMON CHICKEN LEGS

Serves: *4*

Prep Time: *10* Minutes

Cook Time: *50* Minutes

Total Time: 60 Minutes

INGREDIENTS

4 chicken legs
Juice from 1 lemon
2 tablespoons olive oil
1 tsp rosemary
1 tsp seasoning
2 garlic cloves
4-5 lemon slices

DIRECTIONS

1. In a bowl combine lemon juice, rosemary, olive oil, garlic gloves and seasoning

2. Toss the chicken with the marinade and let it marinade for 60 minutes

3. Place the chicken in a baking dish and 4-5 lemon slices along the chicken

4. Roast the chicken at 350 F for 40-50 minutes
5. When ready remove chicken from the oven and serve

CURRIED BEEF

Serves: *4*

Prep Time: *10*   Minutes

Cook Time: *20*   Minutes

Total Time: 30   Minutes

INGREDIENTS

1 lb. olive oil
1 lb. ground beef
1 garlic clove
2 tsp curry powder
1 tsp pepper
1 tsp salt

DIRECTIONS

1. In a skillet heat olive oil and sauté garlic until soft
2. Add the ground beef, pepper, curry powder and salt
3. When ready remove from heat and serve

SAUTEED SHRIMP

Serves: **4-**

Prep Time: **10**   Minutes

Cook Time: **20**   Minutes

Total Time: 30   Minutes

INGREDIENTS

1 tsp olive oil
1 lb. shrimp
1 tablespoon herbes de Provence
1 tsp salt

DIRECTIONS

1. In a skillet heat olive oil
2. Add shrimp, herbes, salt and pepper
3. Cook the shrimp for 3-4 minutes per side
4. When ready remove to a plate and serve

SLOW COOKER BEEF

Serves: **4-6**

Prep Time: **10**   Minutes

Cook Time: **8**   Hours

Total Time: 8   Hours 10 Minutes

INGREDIENTS

2 lb. roast beef
1 cup beef broth
1 cup apple cider vinegar
1 tsp smoked paprika
1 tsp chili powder
1 tsp garlic powder
1 tsp cumin
1 tsp oregano

DIRECTIONS

1. In a bowl combine all spices together
2. Rub the beef with the mixture and let it marinade for 50-60 minutes
3. Place the beef into a slow cooker

4. Add broth, vinegar and cook on low for 7-8 hours

5. When ready remove from the cooker and serve

TURKEY BURGERS

Serves: **4**

Prep Time: **10** Minutes

Cook Time: **20** Minutes

Total Time: 30 Minutes

INGREDIENTS

1 lb. turkey
1 egg

1 tsp salt
1 tsp seasoning
½ cup red onion
1 tablespoon parsley

DIRECTIONS

1. Combine all ingredients together and mix well
2. Form 3-4 patties
3. In a skillet heat olive oil and cook each patty for 4-5 minutes per side
4. When ready remove from heat and serve

BROCCOLI CASSEROLE

Serves: *4*

Prep Time: *10* Minutes

Cook Time: *15* Minutes

Total Time: 25 Minutes

INGREDIENTS

1 onion

2 chicken breasts
2 tablespoons unsalted butter
2 eggs

2 cups cooked rice
2 cups cheese
1 cup parmesan cheese
2 cups cooked broccoli

DIRECTIONS

1. Sauté the veggies and set aside
2. Preheat the oven to 425 F
3. Transfer the sautéed veggies to a baking dish, add remaining ingredients to the baking dish

4. Mix well, add seasoning and place the dish in the oven
5. Bake for 12-15 minutes or until slightly brown
6. When ready remove from the oven and serve

BEAN FRITATTA

Serves: **2**

Prep Time: **10**   Minutes

Cook Time: **20**   Minutes

Total Time: 30   Minutes

INGREDIENTS

1 cup black beans
1 tablespoon olive oil
½ red onion
2 eggs

¼ tsp salt
2 oz. cheddar cheese
1 garlic clove
¼ tsp dill

DIRECTIONS

1. In a bowl whisk eggs with salt and cheese
2. In a frying pan heat olive oil and pour egg mixture
3. Add remaining ingredients and mix well
4. Serve when ready

ROASTED SQUASH

Serves: **3-4**

Prep Time: **10**   Minutes

Cook Time: **20**   Minutes

Total Time: 30   Minutes

INGREDIENTS

2 delicata squashes
2 tablespoons olive oil
1 tsp curry powder
1 tsp salt

DIRECTIONS

1. Preheat the oven to 400 F

2. Cut everything in half lengthwise

3. Toss everything with olive oil and place onto a
    prepared baking sheet

4. Roast for 18-20 minutes at 400 F or until golden
    brown

5. When ready remove from the oven and serve

CUCUMBER CHIPS

Serves: **2**

Prep Time: **10** Minutes

Cook Time: **20** Minutes

Total Time: 30 Minutes

INGREDIENTS

1 lb. cucumber
1 tsp salt
1 tsp smoked paprika
1 tablespoon olive oil

DIRECTIONS

1. Preheat the oven to 425 F
2. In a bowl toss everything with olive oil and seasoning
3. Spread everything onto a prepared baking sheet
4. Bake for 8-10 minutes or until crisp
5. When ready remove from the oven and serve

SQUASH CHIPS

Serves: **2**

Prep Time: **10** Minutes

Cook Time: **20** Minutes

Total Time: 30 Minutes

INGREDIENTS

1 lb. squash
1 tsp salt
1 tsp smoked paprika
1 tablespoon olive oil

DIRECTIONS

1. Preheat the oven to 425 F
2. In a bowl toss everything with olive oil and seasoning
3. Spread everything onto a prepared baking sheet
4. Bake for 8-10 minutes or until crisp
5. When ready remove from the oven and serve

ZUCCHINI CHIPS

Serves: **2**

Prep Time: **10** Minutes

Cook Time: **20** Minutes

Total Time: 30 Minutes

INGREDIENTS

1 lb. zucchini
1 tsp salt
1 tsp smoked paprika
1 tablespoon olive oil

DIRECTIONS

1. Preheat the oven to 425 F
2. In a bowl toss everything with olive oil and seasoning
3. Spread everything onto a prepared baking sheet
4. Bake for 8-10 minutes or until crisp
5. When ready remove from the oven and serve

POTATO CHIPS

Serves: **2**

Prep Time: **10** Minutes

Cook Time: **20** Minutes

Total Time: 30 Minutes

INGREDIENTS

1 lb. potatoes
2 tablespoons olive oil
1 tablespoon smoked paprika
1 tablespoon salt

DIRECTIONS

1. Preheat the oven to 425 F
2. In a bowl toss everything with olive oil and seasoning
3. Spread everything onto a prepared baking sheet
4. Bake for 8-10 minutes or until crisp
5. When ready remove from the oven and serve

PIZZA

ZUCCHINI PIZZA

Serves: **6-8**

Prep Time: **10**   Minutes

Cook Time: **15**   Minutes

Total Time: 25   Minutes

INGREDIENTS

1 pizza crust
½ cup tomato sauce
¼ black pepper
1 cup zucchini slices
1 cup mozzarella cheese
1 cup olives

DIRECTIONS

1. Spread tomato sauce on the pizza crust
2. Place all the toppings on the pizza crust
3. Bake the pizza at 425 F for 12-15 minutes
4. When ready remove pizza from the oven and serve

CAULIFLOWER PIZZA

Serves: **6-8**

Prep Time: **10** Minutes

Cook Time: **15** Minutes

Total Time: 25 Minutes

INGREDIENTS

1 pizza crust
2 oz. parmesan cheese
1 tablespoon olive oil
4-5 basil leaves
1 cup mozzarella cheese
1 cup cauliflower

DIRECTIONS

1. Spread tomato sauce on the pizza crust
2. Place all the toppings on the pizza crust
3. Bake the pizza at 425 F for 12-15 minutes
4. When ready remove pizza from the oven and serve

ARTICHOKE AND SPINACH PIZZA

Serves: **6-8**

Prep Time: **10**   Minutes

Cook Time: **15**   Minutes

Total Time: 25   Minutes

INGREDIENTS

1 pizza crust
1 garlic clove
½ lb. spinach
½ lb. soft cheese
2 oz. artichoke hearts
1 cup mozzarella cheese
1 tablespoon olive oil

DIRECTIONS

1. Spread tomato sauce on the pizza crust
2. Place all the toppings on the pizza crust
3. Bake the pizza at 425 F for 12-15 minutes
4. When ready remove pizza from the oven and serve

MINT PIZZA

Serves: **6-8**

Prep Time: **10**   Minutes

Cook Time: **15**   Minutes

Total Time: 25   Minutes

INGREDIENTS

1 pizza crust
1 olive oil
1 garlic clove
1 cup mozzarella cheese
2 oz. mint
2 courgettes

DIRECTIONS

1. Spread tomato sauce on the pizza crust
2. Place all the toppings on the pizza crust
3. Bake the pizza at 425 F for 12-15 minutes
4. When ready remove pizza from the oven and serve

SAUSAGE PIZZA

Serves: **6-8**

Prep Time: **10**   Minutes

Cook Time: **15**   Minutes

Total Time: 25   Minutes

INGREDIENTS

2 pork sausages
1 tablespoon olive oil
2 garlic cloves
1 tsp fennel seeds
½ lb. ricotta
1 cup mozzarella cheese
1 oz. parmesan cheese
1 pizza crust

DIRECTIONS

1. Spread tomato sauce on the pizza crust
2. Place all the toppings on the pizza crust
3. Bake the pizza at 425 F for 12-15 minutes
4. When ready remove pizza from the oven and serve

HEALTY PIZZA

Serves: **6-8**

Prep Time: **10**   Minutes

Cook Time: **15**   Minutes

Total Time: 25   Minutes

INGREDIENTS

1 pizza crust
1 tablespoon olive oil
1 garlic clove
1 cup tomatoes
1 cup mozzarella cheese
1 carrot

1 cucumber

DIRECTIONS

1. Spread tomato sauce on the pizza crust
2. Place all the toppings on the pizza crust
3. Bake the pizza at 425 F for 12-15 minutes
4. When ready remove pizza from the oven and serve

Conclusion

Your digestive system is a fine balance and keeping it sometimes can be hard to do, but I hope some of the advice in this book can help you gain a healthier digestive system and live a fuller life. Until next time, be happy and be healthy.

www.ingramcontent.com/pod-product-compliance
Lightning Source LLC
Chambersburg PA
CBHW050725030426
42336CB00012B/1420